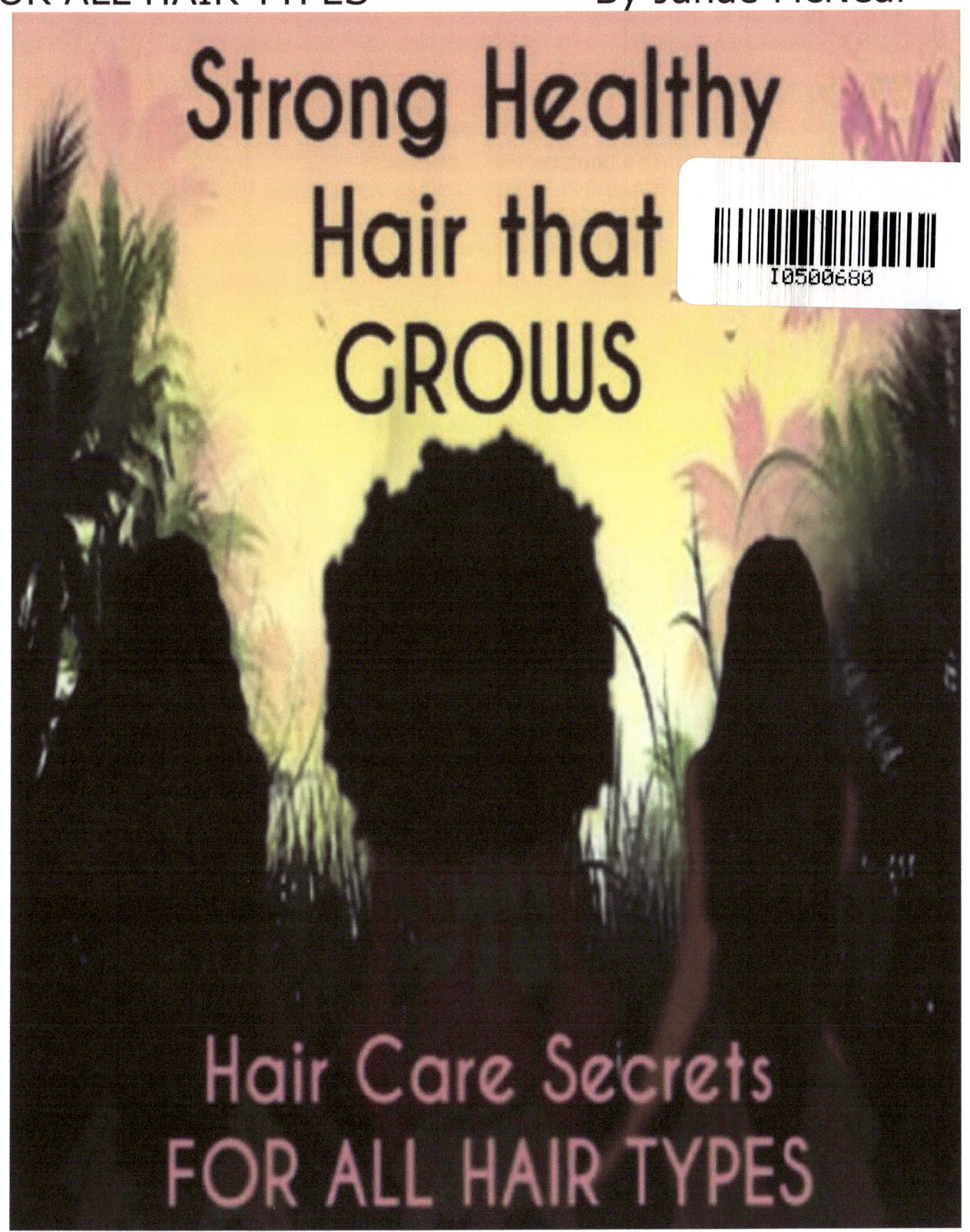

Table of Contents

Dedication

Dedication:

I would like to dedicate this book to my fiancé, Jeremy, and to my dad, Jim, whose constant love and support allow me to follow my dreams.

Chapter 1: Introduction

Hello everyone. I am elated to help you on your journey to longer, stronger, healthier hair. In this book, you will find the results of my research as well as the most successful tips from the trial and error that I have had over the years. I wish something like this was out for me growing up, so I hope you all find new knowledge here that will help you get over a hair stump and lead you to the hair of your dreams.

1-1: My Hair Care Journey

A little about me: I grew up in Atlanta and learned many of the hair myths that some of you may still believe and practice to this day: that using hair grow products that contain petroleum will grow hair, that cutting your ends routinely will make it grow, that brushing your hair a hundred times a day will stimulate hair growth, and that overlapping your relaxers is okay in the name of fashion and can make your hair healthier. These and other harmful hair myths inspired techniques that minimized the growth potential of my hair and caused nothing but damage. I first started receiving relaxers when I was seven years old. Relaxing by itself doesn't have to be damaging, but the way you care for your hair makes all the difference. I didn't know that. When I was a teenager, I experimented with different colors. Color by itself doesn't have to damage the hair, but using it along with relaxers is extremely damaging. I didn't know that.

By the time I was 16, I'd had several types of blonde, two different types of red, black, and even pink hair. When I realized that my hair was irreversibly damaged, I thought I could fix it by dyeing my hair black again. After all, the box said that it would repair my damaged hair, but once damage is done, it's done. It was too late. I would try many things to try and fix the damaged ends without losing inches, including products that claimed to fix split ends and using heat to temporarily mask them, but all that did was damage my hair more.

One notable memory that I have was the day that I was in a perimeter mall in Georgia and a woman came up to me, passed me a card to a beauty salon, and said, "Here, you really need to get rid of all of that damaged hair." She sounded undeniably sarcastic and had a look of disgust on her face when she spoke to me, so I threw the card away thinking she was just in need of an ego trip Even if what she said was true, she wasn't about to get my business. That should have been my turning point, and it propelled me to make some changes, but I defiantly kept my hair after that encounter, thinking that if I just cut the very ends of my hair I would eventually catch up with the split ends without losing too much length. That didn't work.

Once split ends form, they will never stop splitting and will continue to make their way all the way up the hair shaft. It is best to minimize the formation of split ends or you'll have to be strong enough to get rid of them in their entirety if they occur. Letting the majority of your hair go at one time is a difficult experience—enough to make a girl cry. Believe me, I know.

It took several more years of trying to save my already destroyed hair before I had enough. I had lost the battle with my damaged hair. It was time for it to go. I remember the exact day that I decided to shave my head. I was online looking for ways to transition (my first thought was to use transitioning styles and transition from relaxed and colored to natural.) The more I read, the more I realized it would just be much simpler to cut it all off and start over.

I realized after researching that transitioning could potentially be a hit or miss because the point where the old damaged hair meets the new growth is especially weak and prone to more breakage. I decided I didn't want to risk damaging my hair any further or making it harder on myself than it had to be, so I decided to go completely bald. Later on that night, my head was shaved, and I was a new woman. Many people complimented me on my new look, and for a while I contemplated keeping my head shaved. I even started to pick out tattoos, and settled on getting a dragon skull tattoo to complement my new fierce look. It takes a confident woman to be bald in my opinion, and it's not for everybody. Luckily, I have a nice-shaped head.

to miss having long hair. This prompted me to start experimenting with wigs and to research once and for all how to grow my hair and keep it healthy. I found an abundance of information on the subject and began to have many trials and errors from all of the new information that I was sifting through. It was overwhelming at times. Some of the things that I tried flat out didn't work, but many of the things that I learned stuck with me, and I settled into a new improved regimen, unlike anything I had ever done before.

With all of the research and application I was doing, it became clear to me that I had to be more conscious about the products that I was buying from the store and placing into my hair. I tried many products that catered to naturally curly heads but was slightly disappointed every time. It seemed that every product I came across only gave a few of the results that I was expecting. I was looking for one product that strengthened, moisturized, benefited the scalp as much as the hair, was a heat protector, didn't clog my pores, was a growth product, added shine to the hair without being too greasy, protected against damaged ends, and could be used whether I air dried my hair or wanted to wear it straight. I was beginning to get used to having to use several products to achieve the results I was after when a huge light bulb went off in my head.

"Wait a minute," I thought. "Why do I have to settle for barely good enough? Why can't I make my own product that provides everything that I am looking for in one?" I began to research different oils, butters, and herbs that would benefit the hair in all of the ways that I was trying to accomplish. It took me about a year of trial and error to create a product that I was proud of, and my hair began to flourish. Starting out, I was all about what was beneficial to myself and what grew my hair, but others began to take notice. It wasn't long before people started to ask me how I got my hair so thick, why it was growing so fast, and how it remained so healthy. I told them I made my own product and was having these wonderful results, and people began to want to try it.

For a while I was only giving it away to my friends and family, but when they started to have these awesome results as well, I knew I had something amazing on my hands. That's when I decided to make it available to the masses, come up with a company name, and develop a website. If you would like to purchase my product, it is available at

LuBeautyProducts.com. I have gotten nothing but positive feedback from it. It's all natural and full strength, without filler ingredients, which means that it gives the full benefits of every ingredient in it.

I have a wide range of clientele: from men who want to grow their beards to women who want to strengthen and grow their hair. I've had many clients get awesome benefits from my product, many of those who choose to continue to relax their hair. I've even had a client tell me that it soothed and healed a relaxer burn on her scalp and ear within two days. I've been in business for almost two years now, and I love helping people discover new ways to care for their hair. Many who have no clue about their hair, who were just like me, reach their full growth potential.

1-2: The Defining Moment:

The defining moment when I knew I had to write this book was when I was at an event last year. Two young ladies, who I'll call Samantha and Rebecca, were talking about hair. Samantha had been growing her natural hair for quite some time; Rebecca had just done the "big chop" and started over. Rebecca was wearing her natural hair texture dyed a cute blonde color, and it fit her perfectly. I remember thinking that it's okay to dye your hair, even to use other chemicals such as relaxers or texturizers on your hair, if you know how to take care of it afterwards.

I listened to the two women talk about their hair care regimens. Samantha's hair was in twists and probably stopped at the middle of her neck. It was visually a little shorter, but I took into account that she may have had shrinkage. She mentioned she had been growing her hair for almost two years, and I remember thinking her hair could be much longer within that time frame. What Rebecca said next is when I knew I had to write this book.

Samantha asked her what type of products she used. Rebecca replied with a product that she used to grease her hair that was full of petroleum. She also mentioned that she used a brush and gel to make her hair lay down, and I just cringed on the inside. The look that Samantha gave Rebecca indicated that she knew that her hair care regimen was detrimental, but she chose not to comment on her product choices. The first thought that came to my mind was that I hoped she wasn't trying to grow her hair out with those methods. It would be okay if she planned to keep her hair short and colored, but if she ever tried to grow it out, she would be in trouble.

I gave both ladies my business card, chatted with them about some important points on hair care, and wished them the best on their hair care journeys. That instance was the defining moment for me, but it wasn't the only one I had experienced up to that point. There were a plethora of encounters with coworkers, strangers, and friends when I discovered many of them were still holding onto outdated information about hair care. The majority of them couldn't get their hair to grow past a certain level (or at all), and I would help them to the best of my ability, asking them about their regimens and then offering some minor changes that would bring big results.

Many of them would be adamant about their wrong-held convictions, going so far as to state, "Well that's not the way I was taught" or "Those are the products I grew up with" or "That's not how my friend said to grow my hair." Meanwhile, the people who they have been getting advice from weren't able to grow their hair themselves or it took them much longer than it had to. In that instance, I would tell them that they must try something new in order to get new results; some remained stubborn nonetheless and are no better off, unfortunately. I have spent many years studying and researching hair, applying different methods, and sifting through what works and what doesn't work. I am here to present you with the best methods that I have come across and that have been successful on myself, my friends, my family, and customers.

This guide will include what you need to know about growing long, strong, healthy hair. You probably have come to this book because you have either reached a growth plateau, have decided to go natural, have damaged hair, or just want more knowledge about your hair in general. Whatever your reason for reading this book, you will be satisfied with the knowledge that you learn, as there is new knowledge for all audiences. Even if you only decide to apply a few of these methods in your daily regimen, you will notice a positive difference in the way your hair behaves and grows. Nonetheless, to obtain the maximum benefit from this book, I recommend that you use all of the tips provided to create a new regimen for yourself.

Chapter 2: The Science of Hair

In order to grow your hair long, strong, and healthy, you will need know the science behind your hair. Knowing as much about your hair as possible will promote healthy hair care practices in general. Knowing the "why" in hair care will be much more effective than me just listing off a bunch of methods to use. It will make changes in your routine easier for you to accomplish and more natural for you.

If you are anything like me, you will be tempted to skip this section. Why? Because I like to get to the nitty gritty and get my hands dirty. I'm a doer, and I usually like to skip the educational part and get straight to the application. I'm the person that does that over and over with no hesitation and wonder why I have pieces left over when I've put something together incorrectly. You do not want to do that with this book. From what I have learned in the past, you make way too many mistakes that could have been avoided if you were just patient enough to get the educational part out of the way first. I have done years of research and application before writing this book, and I am here to share my full experience with you.

2-1: How Does Hair Grow

First I am going to discuss what hair is made of. In short, hair is made mostly of a protein called keratin. In order to grow, the hair has three main components: the hair bulb, the hair follicle, and the sebaceous gland (also known as the oil gland for short). Diagram 2.1 illustrates these three components. The hair bulb houses the hair follicle, which is where the hair grows. The hair follicle itself can be broken down further into two components: the hair root, which is located below the skin, and the hair shaft, which is the hair you see growing out of your scalp. The oil gland provides nourishment to the hair follicle. Some people's oil glands produces more sebum than others, which is what provides nourishment for the hair and also why they have to wash their hair more often. Too much sebum can leave the hair oily. Some people's oil glands aren't as active, which is why they use other oils to compensate. It is also important to note that your hair texture and pattern will determine how easily oil travels down the hair shaft. The curlier the hair, the harder it is for the natural nutrients to travel from the root to the tip of the hair.

It is important for hair to be moisturized from the root to the tip in order to preserve the hair. Moisture makes hair more elastic, meaning that the hair becomes durable and will stretch more before breaking. Brittle dry hair, the opposite of elastic hair, will cause the hair to break off. Also keep in mind that too much moisture without strength will cause hair to be too soft and break off as well. It is important to have a balance. We will discuss using water and oil to moisturize the hair, which nutrients are necessary for hair growth, and strengthening the hair in later chapters, as moisturizing the hair and making sure it has sufficient nutrients and strength is essential to hair growth.

2-2: The Layers of The Hair Shaft

Now we are going to discuss the hair shaft itself. The hair shaft is made up of three layers: the medulla, the cortex, and the cuticle, listed in order from the innermost layer of hair to the outside of the hair shaft. Diagram 2.2 illustrates these three components. The medulla is thinner or nonexistent in fine hair and strong and prominent in thicker hair. The next layer of the hair is the cortex. This layer makes up the majority of the hair, up to 90%. It is imperative to know how to reach and manipulate the cortex of the hair if you plan to moisturize and strengthen the hair. The last layer of the hair is called the cuticle.

The cuticle is what protects the hair by encasing it. Knowing how to open the hair cuticlewill aid in manipulating the cortex of the hair, moisturizing and strengthening it. Knowing how to close the cuticle will aid in protecting the hair and also add to the shine of the hair. I have included an entire chapter on how to manipulate the cuticle of the hair, as the knowledge is imperative to maximize the benefits that you receive from your hair treatments.

2-3: Hair Growth Phases

The next important topic of discussion is that hair has three growth phases: the anagen, catagen, and telogen phases. The anagen phase is considered the hair's growing phase. This phase usually lasts years (up to seven on average), and most of the hairs on your head are going through this phase at any given time. How much your hair grows is mostly up to genetics (on average half inch a month), but there are ways to manipulate the hair and scalp to maximize its growth potential.

The second phase is called the catagen phase. This phase lasts about a week and a half. The hair follicle shrinks in this phase, and the hair slows down on growth, getting ready for the next phase. This phase is like the fall of hair growth getting ready for a cold, hard winter. The last phase is called the telogen phase. The telogen phase is considered the resting and shedding phase. About 15% of your hair is going through this phase at all times.

It is normal to shed up to 100 hairs a day. Any more than that and you need to figure out what is causing it to shed excessively and change your hair care regimen accordingly. If you are losing more than that in your brushes and combs, then you really have a problem to address if you are trying to grow your hair. The key is to know how each phase affects your hair and to take the necessary measures to promote growth and retain the hair. I often tell people that hair retention is just as important as hair growth. The hair can grow fast, but if it is shedding at a higher rate due to a bad hair care regimen, then you will achieve nothing.

Chapter 3: Scalp Health

In order to grow long, thick, healthy hair, it is imperative to know how to take care of the scalp. The scalp is the foundation, as it is where your hair sprouts from. Think of it like the soil of your garden. The soil needs the correct maintenance and nutrients to grow healthy plants. Many people tend to undervalue how big a role the scalp plays in growing healthy, long hair. Making sure to cover all aspects of the hair care process will ensure maximum results. A damaged, clogged, unhealthy scalp will greatly inhibit the growth and health of your hair. These are the important aspects for keeping a scalp optimal for hair growth.

3-1: Keeping the Scalp Clean

The first important step to keeping a healthy scalp optimal for hair growth is a clean scalp. Regular cleaning keeps the hair follicle and scalp clean and unclogged. The scalp can become clogged with too much product build-up and the build-up of dead skin cells, also known as dandruff. The scalp needs to be thoroughly cleansed; how often you cleanse your scalp will be determined by several factors.

The first factor is how oily your scalp naturally gets. Some people choose to wash their scalps and hair every day because they produce sebum at a faster rate than others. These people usually have no problem growing their hair. Sebum itself is good for hair; people who produce more of it find that they grow their hair quicker than others, but their hair is easily weighed down and becomes too oily. Also, the scalp can become clogged with a mixture of sebum and dead skin cells. If you find that your hair and scalp becomes dry easily, chances are that you produce sebum at a much slower rate. You won't have to wash your hair as often, and should try to use products that mimic the benefits that sebum has for your scalp and hair. You can read more about penetrative oils that mimic the benefits of sebum in the moisturizing chapter.

This brings us to our next point of interest about what determines how often you should be washing your hair and scalp: the type of products that you use. The types of products that you use on your hair factors in on how quickly your scalp and hair follicles become clogged. In a perfect world, I would suggest that you only use natural products that don't clog the scalp and hair, but I know many of you are more concerned about the temporary look of the hair rather than the long-term health. For those that are going to use harsh chemicals regardless, you need to aim to wash your hair a minimum of two times a week, clarifying the hair and scalp at least once a week.

To clarify the hair means to remove the weekly build-up of film that your products are leaving on your hair and scalp. Although this is important whether you are using natural or chemical-laden products, it will be more important if you are regularly use chemicals. If you leave a build-up of products on your hair, it will eventually weigh your hair down and clog your scalp and hair follicles, causing the hair to become harder to manage and prone to damage. You can use an apple cider vinegar rinse to clarify the hair and scalp.

Apple cider vinegar can be found in most grocery stores located next to the white vinegar. It is cheap, usually less than a dollar, and a bottle can last you for months. Make the apple cider vinegar rinse (ACV rinse) by mixing one tablespoon of ACV in a full 700 mL bottle of room temperature water. I find that the water bottles with the sports top work best for me. Using an apple cider vinegar rinse, make sure to thoroughly rub it into the scalp and throughout the hair from root to tip. Apple cider vinegar also has nutrients in it that nourishes the scalp and minimizes dandruff.

Some of you are used to only washing your hair once a week. Even if you only use natural products, I would strongly suggest washing your hair *at least* twice a week—that's the minimum, and that's with minimal product use and sweating, which brings us to our next point: the more you sweat, the more you need to wash your hair. Sweat causes a build-up of dirt, which clogs the pores on your scalp and hair follicles. During the winter months, you could get away with washing your hair less often because you don't sweat as much. I would still recommend washing twice a week during winter.

During the summer, you ideally should wash your hair more often. This will be easier for people with natural hair textures that don't require constant heat to achieve their desired hairstyle. Some weeks during the summer I might even wash my hair every day. Keep in mind that shampoo can dry the hair. If your hair is prone to dryness, I would recommend washing with shampoo at least once a week, and the other times you can co-wash your hair (with conditioner and water only). Make sure to focus on the scalp, not just the hair. It's not necessary to rub conditioner into the scalp, but make sure you massage the scalp with water if you are only co-washing your hair.

I also recommend doing weekly apple cider vinegar rinses, where you massage it into your entire scalp and rub it gently downward through your hair to your tips. During the summer, it is easy to wear a wash and go style, meaning sometimes I just wash my hair, towel dry it, moisturize it, throw it in a ponytail or put a cute headband on, and let it air dry in its natural pattern. Wash and go styles can be beneficial to your hair, causing it to flourish. Now that you know all of the benefits of keeping a clean scalp, we will talk about the next point of interest:

3-2: Providing Necessary Nutrients

Providing the scalp with beneficial nutrients to support healthy hair growth can make or break your hair. Creating an optimal scalp environment by adding the necessary nutrients will maximize growth potential. You can do this topically and through your diet. Getting enough of vitamins A, B, C, D, and E; iron; zinc; and magnesium will help you reach maximum growth potential. It is best to get them in your diet through food or supplements with added vitamins in your hair care products to gain even more benefits from them.

Something else you should get plenty of in your diet is protein. The majority of hair is made of protein, so it only makes sense that eating plenty of it and doing protein treatments on your hair will help you grow it long, strong, and healthy. Be careful with protein treatments though because having them too often will cause hair to break off, especially if it isn't balanced with the right amount of moisture. I go in depth about protein treatments in Chapter 6.

3-3: Added Ways to Control Dandruff

One last important thing I'd like to mention about scalp health is an added way to control the accumulation of dead skin cells, also known as dandruff. It is important to mention that no product will be able to take the place of properly cleansing the scalp and hair regularly, but if you have dandruff build-up in spite of proper cleaning, this method may prove successful for you. The use of coconut oil has many benefits, and one notable one for the scalp besides moisturizing is that it has anti-microbial properties. This can help with keeping dandruff at bay and creates an optimal scalp environment most suitable for growing the hair. My products contain coconut oil for this very reason.

Apple cider vinegar rinses are known to keep dandruff at bay for this reason as well. Now you know how scalp health plays a role in growing healthy, long, strong hair and have all of the information about scalp health that you need to reach the maximum benefits of your hair goals. This information alone will cause a noticeable difference in the health of your hair, but we are just getting started. There's a lot more information to cover.

Chapter 4: Manipulating the Hair Cuticle and Why it's Important

Before we get into moisturizing, strengthening, and growing the hair, I thought it was imperative to talk about how to manipulate the hair strand, mainly the hair cuticle, to maximize the rewards of your hair care regimens. This knowledge will be extremely helpful, as your efforts to penetrate your hair with your preferred treatments won't be hit or miss. Sure, you could have some success without applying the following methods, but applying this information will save you money and time and will make everything you do to your hair have a much greater impact. In other words, you won't have to use as much product and take as much time doing your treatments if you use the following methods correctly.

4-1: Methods to Open the Hair Cuticle

The cuticle of the hair protects the medulla and the cortex. The cortex of the hair makes up the majority of the strand, and when you apply products and treatments, you are trying to manipulate the cortex. In order to have the greatest effect of the cortex, you will have to learn how to open the cuticle of the hair without damaging the hair and also know how to close the cuticle when you are done to protect everything that you are trying to accomplish. If the cuticle of the hair is closed while you try to apply your products, a minimum amount of the product will absorb into the hair. If the cuticle is left open after you apply your products, most of the product will escape the hair and you will have to apply the products more often.

As shown in diagram 4.1, the cuticle of the hair looks like a shingled roof that can be raised and lowered. These are my two favorite methods that I regularly use to open the hair cuticle. Deliberately opening the cuticle before applying your products and treatments will ensure that the maximum amount is absorbed into your hair. This is my preferred method, as it is extremely effective: good old baking soda. Baking soda is actually known to replaced shampoo altogether with it. I prefer to use it only before applying my hair treatments because it doesn't lather.

To use baking soda to open the hair cuticle and prime your hair before your hair treatments, mix a teaspoon of baking soda in a full 700 mL bottle of warm water. You can buy and reuse bottled water with a sports top; that's what I use, and it makes the application easier. Shake the contents of the bottle until the baking soda is completely dissolved to ensure uniform application. Squirt the baking soda mixture through your entire head of hair from root to tip. Try not to rub your hair too much, as you may accidently close the hair cuticle by rubbing your hair in a downward motion.

I usually go on to apply my treatments, waiting to wash it out only after I finish them, but if you have sensitive skin, I would suggest rinsing the baking soda mixture out of your hair with warm water prior to your other treatments. Make sure not to rub the hair too much while doing this because rubbing the hair downward can close the hair cuticle. Rubbing the hair upward will not aid in opening the cuticle; it could actually be damaging to your hair by causing too much unnecessary friction. Your cuticle will now be open and ready for you to apply your hair treatments. You can use this method before deep conditioning, henna, and protein treatments, and it will ensure that the maximum amount of the treatment is absorbed into your hair.

The reason why baking soda works to open the cuticle is because baking soda is a base. A base will raise the cuticle of the hair. Baking soda is the only base I will mention as it is the only one I have used with success on my hair. Keep in mind that I wouldn't recommend using more than a teaspoon dissolved in a full 700 mL bottle of warm water.

The second method I will discuss to open the hair cuticle is good old plain warm water. The water should be warmer than lukewarm, but be careful that it is not too hot or you could burn yourself. Also keep in mind that too much heat applied to the hair can damage the hair, especially the ends. Heat will open the hair cuticle, although I find that the baking soda method does a much better job at it. Using heat to open the hair cuticle explains why people find that sitting under a hair dryer works better when doing hair treatments. Now you know the science behind it; it is because it keeps the hair cuticle open. If your hair and skin are sensitive, I would recommend using this method instead of the baking soda method. Even if you decide to use the baking soda method as your preferred method, you can use this knowledge during the duration of your hair treatments. Now you know your treatments will absorb better if you keep the hair warm by either sitting under the dryer with a plastic cap or wrapping a towel around your plastic cap to trap warmth in your hair.

4-2: Methods to Close the Hair Cuticle:

Now that you know how to successfully open the hair cuticle, I am going to explain to you how to close it. It is critical to close the hair cuticle after you have finished your treatments. The cuticle of your hair is what protects the cortex and the medulla and makes sure that moisture doesn't escape from your hair. Leaving the cuticle open will be detrimental to your hair, causing it to become dry, easier to damage, and look dull instead of shiny.

My preferred method of closing the hair cuticle is to use apple cider vinegar. Acids, which are the opposite of bases, have the ability to close the hair cuticle. Apple cider vinegar is naturally acidic, and when diluted properly with water, has many benefits to the hair. Along with closing the cuticle of the hair, apple cider vinegar has vitamins in it that nourish the scalp and hair and can eliminate dandruff and an itchy scalp because of its antimicrobial properties. It causes hair to shine and to retain moisture better. Many of you may be worried about the smell that vinegar will leave in your hair, but do not fret, the smell amazingly disappears when your hair dries.

I mix one tablespoon of apple cider vinegar into afull 700 mL bottle of room temperature water. Cold water is fine too; just make sure the water isn't warm as warm water will encourage the hair cuticle to remain open. Shake the mixture to ensure uniform application throughout your hair. After applying, it is okay to rub it gently into your scalp and through your hair downwards, all the way through your ends. Make sure to be gentle, especially with the ends of your hair. For most people, it isn't necessary to rinse the vinegar mix out of your hair after application; you can just let it dry in your hair. For those that may be extremely sensitive to the vinegar, you can try rinsing the mixture out with cold water after application, if you still find yourself sensitive to this mixture, this next method may be for you.

The next method is plain cold water. You may have heard that cold water will improve the shininess of your hair, and now you know why. It is because cold water naturally closes the cuticle of your hair. It is also why some people will dry their hair with cold air the last few minutes of drying it. I find that the added benefits of apple cider vinegar make it my preferred method, but in a pinch, using cold water will work as well.

4-3: Side Notes:

As I mentioned before, some people swear by the baking soda and water mixture to cleanse your hair. I would suggest to these people that they need to balance the pH of their hair afterwards; leaving the cuticle of your hair open isn't good, especially if you are doing it regularly. You will notice your hair will always be dry because moisture will regularly escape your hair. It also makes your hair prone to damage, as the cortex of the hair will be exposed.

Some people on the other end of the spectrum choose to only use the apple cider vinegar mixture to cleanse the hair. I prefer for my shampoos to lather, so I don't use this method solely for that purpose. An added bonus of baking soda and apple cider vinegar is that they both clarify your hair, meaning that they both remove the added buildup of products that you use every day. This is why I don't worry about chemicals such as sulfates because at least once a week, whether I'm doing hair treatments that week or not, I clarify my hair with the apple cider vinegar mixture. The only time I prefer to use the baking soda mixture is when I'm purposely trying to open my hair cuticle before treatments.

Chapter 5: Moisturizing the Hair

Now that you know how to open the hair cuticle, I will discuss an important part of the hair care process: moisturizing the hair. In order to keep the hair healthy, it needs to retain a great deal or moisture. Regularly moisturizing the hair will improve the elasticity of the hair, reduce the occurrence of split ends, and keep it from breaking off. Remember that moisturizing and strengthening are equally important. Moisture without strength with cause the hair to be too soft and to break off. Strength without moisture will cause the hair to become too dry and break off. It's imperative to keep the correct balance. I will talk about strengthening the hair in the next chapter.

There are several ways to moisturize the hair, which may even challenge some of your beliefs and traditions about hair care, as it did mine when I discovered this information years ago. I had to ditch many hair products that I grew up using and felt downright violated and upset when I found out I had been fooled all those years with products that were misleading. That is the reason I decided to make my own products that do what they actually claim to do. There are no fillers (inactive) ingredients in my products. You can buy my products at LuBeautyProducts.com. They has proven ingredients that are good for the entire head, from your scalp to the tips of your hair.

You have to be careful with products that claim to moisturize the hair because many products use ingredients that only give the appearance of moisture. I say this because many products make the hair slick on the outside but do not actually penetrate the hair. This is why it applies like a greasy film and makes the hair feel weighed down. A product that truly penetrates the hair will moisturize without leaving a film of grease on the outside on the hair. You should choose products that penetrate the hair shaft, moisturizing all of the layers of the hair, not just sitting on top of the products and read the ingredients list. Knowing which substances actually penetrate the hair will help you become more discerning about the products that you buy.

5-1: A Moisturizing Powerhouse

Before we get into the many benefits of oils, I am going to talk about one moisturizer that many people don't give enough credit to: water. Water is actually a good way to moisturize your hair, and it's free. All water isn't created equal though; some water can be harsh on hair. This water is called hard water and should be avoided. Hard water has minerals in it that will dry, damage, and weigh down the hair over time, so you should not use it to wash your hair if you intend to maximize your hair's growth potential. The awful thing is that many states have hard water, and I have included diagram 5.1, which illustrates the hardness levels of the water in each US state.

If you live in a state that has soft water, then congratulations; that is one less thing that you have to worry about. If you live in a state that has hard water, it will cost you a little extra as you will have to buy filtered water from the store to wash your hair or buy a water filter to use at home. The good thing is that it's cheap to obtain filtered water, and it will pay off for you in the long run. The water you use is important because some minerals dry the hair and cause it to be brittle. Brittle hair will eventually become damaged and break off. If you have been using hard water on your hair, you will usually see a big improvement just by switching your water. Still, this is only the beginning; there is much more that needs to be done to maintain a healthy head of hair.

One important thing to note is that although water is a good moisturizer for your hair, how well your hair retains water will be determined by how porous your hair is. The more porous it is, the less it will retain water and penetrative oils. If you notice that you barely have to moisturize your hair, then your hair has a low porosity. These hair types need less moisture than others, and their hair can become weighed down easily. It you notice that your hair dries out fast, then more than likely your hair is highly porous; in other words, moisture can easily escape from your hair. I happen to have naturally porous hair. Some chemicals can make your hair more porous as well, such as relaxers, because they break down the natural protection of your hair. The good thing is that there are a couple of effective methods to counteract porous hair. I will discuss a short-term method for counteracting porous hair in this chapter by using sealant oils. For a more long-term solution, read the strengthening chapter of this book.

5-2: Maximizing Your Benefits from Oils

We have discussed the importance of water for moisturizing hair; now we are going to discuss oils. Although water is a good moisturizer, for those with more porous hair, it's advisable for you to use oil-based moisturizers that are able to cling to your hair better. All oils used to moisturize the hair aren't created equal. Some oils will penetrate the hair shaft better than others.

Some examples of oils that will penetrate the hair quite well are coconut oil, olive oil, avocado oil, shea butter, argan oil, and wheat germ oil. Some natural oils are good for your hair, but only as a sealant, meaning they don't penetrate the hair as well; they are good to protect the outside of the hair by keeping moisture in. Some examples of sealant oils are castor oil, jojoba oil, and grapeseed oil. When applying these oils, you would use your penetrative oil first, then use a sealant oil on top. I highly recommend using natural oils; you will notice a tremendous difference in the health of your hair when you do.

5-3: The Enemy of Healthy Growing Hair

One of the worst things you can put on your hair is petroleum. Another substance you should look out for is petrolatum which is a derivative of petroleum. Many African American products have been using this for years because it is cheap to produce. Even some of your favorite growth products have been using this. I dare you to look at the ingredients list. It doesn't penetrate hair at all. It gives the appearance of moisturizing the outside of the hair but does nothing for the inside of the hair. This is why some of you using these products are unable to grow your hair no matter how hard you try. Not only does it not penetrate the hair, it clogs the scalp, reducing growth potential.

Another important thing to look for is products that claim to be good for you because they have a natural ingredient in them. I won't name any look at the ingredients list. The ingredients list will always name ingredients from most to least; if an ingredients list has petroleum as the first ingredient and coconut oil as the second ingredient, the product could very well contain 99.9% petroleum and .1% coconut oil. Although this product technically has coconut oil in it, that doesn't mean that it contains enough of the active ingredient to have a positive impact on your hair. In this case, the product is being misleading by making you think the .1% of coconut oil will outweigh the negative benefits of the prominent filler ingredient: petroleum.

A filler ingredient is what white bread is to your diet. It is cheap and will fill you up, but it doesn't have much nutritional value. Companies use filler ingredients because they make a product cheap to produce but don't add much value to you as a consumer. This is what led me to make a product that wasn't misleading. All of the ingredients in my product penetrate the hair and scalp, are all natural, and are full strength. Every single one serves a specific purpose for the health of the scalp and hair, from root to tip.

4-4:   Deep Conditioning the Hair:

Now we are going to discuss the importance of deep conditioning the hair. Taking time out of your schedule to deep condition your hair periodically is just as important as the daily moisturizing methods that I have shared with you. Deep conditioning is especially important after doing certain hair treatments such as protein and henna treatments. Starting off, I would recommend doing a deep condition treatment once a week in order to keep the hair in tip-top shape.

Deep conditioning greatly improves the elasticity of the hair, causing a reduction in the occurrence of split ends. Improving the elasticity of the hair improves its breaking point, which means that it can endure harsher handling before it breaks off, compared to dry, brittle hair. You can buy treatments from the store specifically formulated for deep conditioning or you can make your own at home. I like to make mine this way: I heat ¼ cup coconut oil and ¼ cup olive oil on low heat in a small sauce pan. Next, I take a cup of moisturizing conditioner, any specially formulated to moisturize the hair is fine, and add the three ingredients together in a bowl.

This amount works well for my hair, which is mid-back in length. If you need more, you could double up the mixture. It is fine to leave what you have left over in the fridge with a tight lid on it. For your next session, you would just carefully steep the mixture in hot water to rewarm it. I wouldn't recommend microwaving this mixture to reheat it.

Thoroughly coat your hair with the warm mixture and place a plastic cap over your hair. Next, either wrap a towel around your hair or sit under a dryer. Sitting under a dryer would provide the maximum benefit in the shortest amount of time. You should usually deep condition your hair for no less than one hour. When I do my other hair treatments in conjunction with deep conditioning, I let my deep conditioning treatment sit it for a minimum of two hours. After rinsing the treatment out of my hair, I use an apple cider vinegar rinse to close my hair cuticle. You could also do a quick cold rinse on your hair to get the same benefit.

Chapter 6: Strengthening the Hair

Strengthening the hair is just as important as moisturizing the hair. I like to think of myself as a chemist when it comes to hair. You have to strike the right balance between the two. In this section I will talk in depth about the different methods that I use to strengthen my hair.

6-1:   The Perfect Hair Strengthener:

The most important method to strengthen the hair is to add protein to it, as that is what the majority of your hair is made of. You can do this by adding more protein into your diet by eating more meat, lentils, fish, yogurt, cheese, and nuts. You can also do so topically by using protein in your hair treatments. You can buy protein treatments from the store if you prefer, but I'm going to discuss a way to make your protein treatments at home that let you control the ingredients that you put into it. It will be cheaper too.

When many people think of an at-home protein treatment, they automatically think about eggs. The problem with using eggs is that an egg protein is larger than a hair protein, so it doesn't penetrate as well as you would expect. This is why most people using eggs as a protein treatment don't see much of a long-term difference. I was one of these people. I saw the benefits of an egg protein treatment for a maximum of two days before my hair became weak again.

The key is to use a smaller protein that can mimic a hair protein. The most effective at-home method that I have used is gelatin. Gelatin is the same thing they use to make flavored jello. You can find plain, unflavored gelatin on most baking aisles located next to the flavored jellos. The reason why plain gelatin is a great protein treatment is because it contains hydrolyzed proteins, small proteins that will actually penetrate the hair fully.

You can create your protein treatment this way: I place one cup of boiled water in a heat-safe container and add two packets of unflavored gelatin to it, stirring constantly to dissolve it evenly. Once the gelatin is dissolved into the water, cover the container tightly and let it sit until it thickens. Once it thickens, you can add a cheap moisturizing conditioner to it to give it a better consistency. Put this mixture thoroughly through your hair and put a plastic cap on your hair to contain your body heat. You can then wrap a towel around your plastic cap; this will keep your hair warmer, which will improve the absorption of the protein treatment because heat causes the cuticle of the hair to stay open. If you want to sit under a dryer, you can do this as well while wearing the plastic cap.

Never do a gelatin treatment and leave it in your hair without covering it with plastic. I had to learn this the hard way when my head became hard as a rock one day when I ran out of plastic head caps but decided to do the treatment anyways. I freaked out, thinking that I was going to have to cut my hair off again; it was hard like a helmet. It took an eternity, but luckily I was able to wash it out of my hair with hot water.

It is not necessary to leave this mixture on your hair for more than one hour; the protein treatment will have absorbed by then. Rinse the hair thoroughly, first with warm water only, then wash with a shampoo, also with warm water. If protein is the only treatment that you have planned for the day, you will want to deep condition the hair for at least another hour, but more if you have the time. I have included my deep conditioning method in the moisturizing chapter of this book.

Regular protein treatments will strengthen the hair. The amount of protein your hair needs varies from person to person. If you have thick, natural hair, you can start off doing your protein treatments once a month or once every six weeks. If you have weak hair, I suggest using a protein treatment bi-weekly for the first month. You should notice a drastic improvement in your hair's strength after the first two treatments. Then, you can cut back to once a month or every six weeks. Once again, everyone's hair varies; you will have to play around with your own hair to see how much protein is suitable for your individual head. If you see that your hair loses strength quickly, you may want to increase the frequency of protein treatments. Do keep in mind that protein is good for the hair, but too much of it will make your hair brittle, as protein dries out the hair. Brittle hair will break off just like weak hair will, so too much of a good thing could destroy your hair. After every protein treatment, you will need to moisturize the hair thoroughly with a deep conditioning treatment. Never skip this step. Your hair will thank you.

4-2: The Perfect Hair Strengthener's Ally:

I will now discuss another way to strengthen the hair. This is one of my personal favorites. Keep in mind that you shouldn't skip protein treatments altogether while using this method. Using protein is an important part of hair care that shouldn't be skipped, but this method used with protein will greatly improve your hair. All hair textures can benefit from this method, but if you use chemicals to alter your hair texture or color, this method will be even more effective for you. My personal favorite is the use of an herb called henna. You can buy henna at most Indian markets, or if you are unable to find some in your area, you can buy it online. The best way to make sure you are getting pure henna is to buy body art quality (BAQ) henna. This ensures that the henna isn't mixed with harsh chemicals, which is sometimes the case. Once you buy a bag, it will last a while. Depending on your hair length, it can last a few months or more.

I'm a big advocate of henna because it is natural and it improves the elasticity and strength of your hair. It does this by attaching to the protein, which in turn reinforces it. It can also loosen the curl pattern of your hair because it weighs the hair down. Another benefit is that it improves the shine of the hair and strengthens the cuticle as well as the cortex. Henna also pigments the hair red, which is more noticeable in lighter hair colors. This could be a good or a bad thing according to the individual. The more you use it, the darker the color will be because of the build-up of henna on the hair. In darker hair colors, you will notice a red tinge to the hair that is most noticeable in light.

If you have a problem with pigmenting the hair red, you could use an alternative to henna called cassia obovata. It is also an herb that has many of the same properties as henna without the pigment. Many people call it the "colorless henna." I haven't used colorless henna, as I don't mind the slightly red pigment that henna gives my hair, but there is an abundance of research that suggests that it is has many of the same benefits of henna without adding henna's iconic red color.

How to use henna to strengthen the hair: I use about one cup of boiled water to half a cup of henna because I like the consistency. When mixed, it gives the consistency of pudding. This to me, makes the henna easier to work with, as henna can be a messy process. You will want to wear gloves while working with henna, as the dye can stain your hands. I get about 20 pairs for less than a dollar at a dollar store.

Some people like to let their henna sit for hours before application in order to release the dye more, but this isn't necessary if you are only trying to strengthen the hair. If using it to strengthen the hair only, just wait until it cools before you apply it. I often mix my henna with a cheap moisturizing conditioner. It will keep the hair from becoming too dry and will also improve the application experience. Your first time applying henna, you may want to put some dark colored old towels on the floor until you get the hang of it. The dye in it can stain fabrics and other surfaces, such as floors and doors (yes, doors, I still have the frame to prove it!).

Part your hair in sections; four will suffice. Starting in the back and working your way to the front, coat your hair thoroughly with the henna mixture, using your gloved hand or an application brush. Make sure to coat your hair from the root to the tip so your ends are fully saturated. Finally, place a plastic cap on your head. You can then place a dark towel around the plastic cap to keep the hair warm.

The only downside to henna is how long it needs to sit on your hair. I usually let mine sit between four to six hours. On the days that I decide to apply henna, I make sure that I have nothing else to do that day. Another possibility is to leave it in overnight. Leaving it in overnight has the potential to be messy though, as it may seep out depending on how you sleep or if your mixture is too watery. I sleep wildly, so I try to avoid leaving it in while I'm sleeping.

Usually, on the days that I decide to do my henna treatments, I aim to do it on the same day that I do my protein and deep conditioning treatments. You would do the gelatin treatment first, then the henna treatment, then the deep conditioning treatment last. On the days that you do a protein and henna treatment, you would want to leave the deep conditioning treatment in for a much longer time because henna has some of the same effects as protein; it dries your hair. I would recommend at least two hours or more if you can. I repeat, never do a henna or protein treatment without a deep conditioning afterwards. If you don't have time to deep condition afterwards, then you might as well hold off on the whole process until you have the time.

When you first start your henna treatments, you can start to do them weekly for the first month and then decrease to monthly or to every six weeks. You will notice your hair will become stronger and shed less if you strike the right balance of protein, henna, and moisture treatments. You will also see that split ends do not form as easily on the ends of your hair.

Chapter 7: How to Handle the Hair Properly

In this chapter, I'm going to discuss how to handle your hair. The way you handle your hair can make or break it. Many people want to grow their hair long, but it suffers from mistreatment. Mistreatment of the hair can lead to excessive shedding and damage to the hair, creating split ends. Throughout this chapter you may find some myths dispelled about how you thought you should handle your hair.

7-1: General Treatment of the Hair:

The first thing I'm going to discuss is the general treatment some of you use on your hair. Many of you, especially those of you with hair textures that you deemharder to manage, assume that just because your hair texture is kinkier than another hair texture means that it is more durable to the way that you handle your hair, but that is absolutely not true. In fact, kinkier hair usually requires gentler care because of the curl pattern. Every bend in your hair is a potential breaking point, which means you need to be more careful when handling curly and kinky hair textures.

Finer and thinner hair is usually weaker, has a less prominent medulla than other hair textures, and can be found in all hair textures. You can have a head full of curly hair, thinking that your hair is stronger than someone with straight hair, but both of you may have fine hair textures. The same can be applied to thick hair: it can be found in all hair textures, no matter how curly or straight the hair is. Kinkier hair also needs gentler love and care in regards to moisture and strengthening treatments.

In other words, just because you consider your hair as hard to manage doesn't mean that you can yank away at your hair with combs and brushes without damaging it. Usually, the reverse is true. You need to be gentler with these hair types because they are usually more prone to breakage and damage. All hair is like a delicate fabric. You wouldn't iron certain fabrics on a high temperature or relentlessly yank at the fabric, as it would cause it to unravel. You should use this mindset at all times when dealing with your hair.

7-2: The Tools to Use (And Not to Use) on Your Hair:

Now that we have gotten that out of the way, I am going to discuss the tools that you should and shouldn't use on your hair. I see many people who are more concerned with styling the hair than heal it. I see many people using medieval torture methods on their hair in the name of fashion. There is nothing wrong with styling your hair a certain way, but be mindful of the techniques that you use to achieve the style.

Many people style their hair with no regard for the health of their hair and then try to backtrack to fix damage that has already been done. Then they become more concerned with making it look healthy than actually making it healthy (creating split ends and then trying to disguise them later). It's easy to disguise split ends for a short time, but once split ends form they will never go away. The split ends will eventually make their way up the entire hair shaft if you let them remain on your hair.

The only logical method, if you want to grow your hair long and healthy, is to minimize the creation of split ends. The ends of your hair are the oldest part of your hair and will require the most care. When choosing tools for your hair care regimen, you need to get tools that will minimize the stress caused to the ends of your hair. You should also aim to get tools that won't pull out unnecessary strands of your hair. If you are losing a ball of hair every time you style your hair, you need to address why this is happening.

Personally, I will not use any type of brush on my hair, not even a paddle brush. I just feel that it adds too much unnecessary stress to my hair. If you do decide to use one, I would say to use one only if you absolutely must, perhaps just to wrap the hair, and be gentle. Bristle brushes are flat out the wrong type of brush to use unless you have naturally straight and thick hair. If you have a curl pattern of any kind or any type of chemical in your hair (color, relaxer, perm, etc.), you shouldn't use a bristle brush at all unless your intention is to keep your hair buzz-cut short. Bristle brushes are extremely damaging and likely to increase the occurrence of split ends on the wrong hair textures.

So what does that leave you to use on your hair? This brings us to my favorite hair tool: a wooden comb. I gave up using plastic combs altogether when I found out the potential danger that they pose to my hair. The reason you will never see me using a plastic comb on my hair is that they tend to have seams on the comb that tear out unnecessary hair and cause unnecessary split ends. Diagram 7.2 illustrates where the seams are usually found on a comb. There are seamless plastic combs out on the market now, but I won't recommend them, as I haven't used them and don't know of anyone who uses them with success.

The only types of combs that I use on my hair are wooden combs, and they vary from wide tooth to small tooth combs. When I use a wooden comb on my hair, I notice less friction, and the amount of hairs that come out while combing are minimal. Also, many wooden combs come infused with oils that are beneficial to your hair. The best way to detangle your hair would be to start with a wide tooth wooden comb on the very ends of your hair and carefully work your way up. You don't want to comb straight from the root to the tip if there are tangles in your hair because you will pull out extra hair unnecessarily.

Start at the tips, and when you are satisfied that you have removed all of the tangles, you can work your way to the top. Next, take a smaller-tooth comb and do the same thing, working your way up until you are satisfied that you have removed all of the tangles. Then you can gently comb from the root to the tip to make sure all of the tangles have been removed. If you notice some tangles still remain, gently work them out before combing from the root to the tip again. Some people differ on whether they believe you should only comb the hair when it's wet or dry. I personally aim to only comb my hair while it's wet and slippery with conditioner in it. This makes sure that the hair is elastic and less likely to break off. I've also noticed that my hair's natural disposition is to like as much water as possible.

After combing, I plait it or twist it so that it doesn't re-tangle while it dries. Four plaits or twists—two in the front, two in the back—will suffice. I air dry my hair as much as possible, only using a hand dryer or sitting under a dryer unless it's an emergency. Sitting under a dryer is better for your hair because it distributes heat evenly, and it is best to invest in one to use at home. When using a hand dryer, make sure to use only medium heat and dry the hair in sections. Don't hold the dryer directly on the hair; although your hair will dry faster, it can damage your hair.

If I plan to straighten my hair, I will comb it while it is dry because I have to, but I make sure that my hair is thoroughly moisturized from the root to the tip, a little more so since I'm about to apply heat on it, in sections, and I am extremely careful and gentle with my hair at all times. I use a hot iron with pure ceramic plates. Using ceramic plates are less damaging on the hair because they distribute heat evenly and prevent cold and hot spots. Be careful because some flat irons say that they are ceramic but are only ceramic coated over metal. Make sure that the flat iron states that it is ceramic all the way through. I will not use heat above 400 degrees on my hair, and the product that I use (my product) to protect my hair is a moisturizer, strengthener, and heat protector in one. It was carefully formulated with your entire head in mind, from your scalp health to the ends of your hair.

7-3: How to Wash Your Hair:
Next I'm going to discuss how to properly wash and clean the hair. I am going to discuss my regimen and tell you why I feel that it is successful; it may challenge some of the things that you already know. How often you wash your hair will in part be determined by how busy you are, what type of products you use on your hair, and your hair's disposition to water. Regardless of this, you should aim to wash your hair at least twice a week. This is to keep the scalp unclogged and the hair clean. You may wash it more depending on the type of products you use, the time of year, and how much sebum oil your scalp naturally produces.

I previously discussed, in the moisturizing chapter of this book, the importance of using the correct type of water for your hair, and I included a water map of the US that describes where hard water and soft water can be found. If you live where there is hard water, I strongly recommend getting a water filter or buying filtered water from the store to wash your hair. Hard water contains minerals that are drying to the hair and can cause damage. I know many people are extremely picky about the shampoo and conditioners sulfates, but you won't find me among them. I like for my shampoos to lather, so I am satisfied buying regular shampoos and conditioners, as long as they are moisturizing to the hair.

In a pinch, I'll even use Suave Naturals. I've used the expensive shampoos and conditioners on my hair, and I haven't noticed anything that I can't replicate at home for a lower price. For instance, I know some people won't use certain shampoos and conditioners for fear of build-up on their hair. I remedy that by using a weekly apple cider vinegar rinse to clarify the hair.

After thoroughly washing the hair, lightly wring the extra moisture out of your hair and wrap it in a microfiber towel. You don't want to use a traditional towel because a little known fact is that traditional towels can strip your hair of needed moisture. Furthermore, the material that most towels are made of can cause friction causing you hair to split. I use a Turbi Twist towel, but any microfiber towel will work just fine.

7-4:   How and When to Trim Your Ends:

Growing up, I believed the myth that somehow trimming the ends of my hair would inspire my scalp to produce more hair. This seemed to be a myth that was running rampant among my friends and family. This myth is simply untrue. Cutting the ends of your hair does not dictate how much your hair grows in any capacity. The only things that determine how much your hair grows is your diet, your genetics, and the health of your scalp and hair follicle.

Hair grows about half an inch on average; it can be more or less depending on your genetics and the way you take care of it. Imagine if your hair grows half an inch a month and your schedule is to cut your hair a quarter inch or more a month. With that schedule you will barely see any results from your hard work. Instead, you need to learn to recognize a split end. Diagram 7.4 demonstrates what a healthy hair looks like compared to what a split end looks like.

The only time the ends of your hair need to be cut is if split ends have developed. Now you see why I say that reducing the development of split ends is more important that trying to disguise or cut split ends once they form. The more you are diligent in your hair care regimen to minimize the occurrence of split ends, the less you have to cut your hair and the more growth you will see. Instead of cutting your hair on a schedule, cut it on a need-to basis.

You can cut your ends at home; make sure to use sharp scissors made specifically for cutting hair. If you don't feel confident enough to do it at home, then let a professional do it. I am wary of letting someone else cut my hair because I am a control freak and don't like putting the fate of my hair in a stranger's hands who may be too trim-happy. I choose to cut my ends at home and just snip split ends as they form.

7-5: Different Materials and How They Affect Your Hair:

When I was younger, I thought I was doing right by wrapping my hair and tying it up every night with a scarf. My intentions were good; the only problem is that I was using a cotton scarf. My hair probably would have had a better chance if I had just left it untied instead of using cotton to tie my hair. The fabric that you use to tie your hair up with is extremely important because some fabrics are better at retaining moisture than others.

Cotton happens to be one of the worst, as it draws moisture away from your hair, causing it to dry out. Many of you are already aware of this because satin caps have become popular. I even see many women wearing them out in public. The reason why satin is a better choice is because it helps retain moisture inside of the hair without absorbing much into the fabric. For this reason, satin is a good cost-effective method for protecting the hair at night and keeping it moisturized.

Satin is good, but my absolute favorite is silk. I noticed ten times more benefits after I started using my silk cap. I noticed that silk doesn't allow any moisture to escape from my hair at all. Also, silk is an extremely smooth fabric—much smoother than satin—that doesn't cause any friction to the hair, which is important because it doesn't cause split ends. I also noticed that my satin caps start to get runs in them and have to be replaced often in order to keep the same benefits. I haven't had any problems with my silk cap; no matter how much I use it and wash it it's still in perfect condition.

Silk is a little pricier, but it's worth it. I bought my silk cap on Amazon, and it is specifically made for longer hair. It fits like an enclosed durag and was made with 100% Indian silk. Be careful to get genuine 100% silk; manmade silk won't have the same benefits.

If you are the type that doesn't like to tie your hair up at night for whatever reason—maybe it is uncomfortable for you or the hubby can't stand the sight of it—this method is definitely for you. Use satin or silk bedding. I would recommend silk once again, but silk can get a little pricy, especially for a full bed set. It is worth the investment if you can do it, but satin would be the next best thing.

Regardless of whether I decide to use a cap or depend on my bedding that night, I always put my hair in two plaits before going to bed. This ensures that your hair won't tangle as much overnight for those who sleep wild like I do. For those with straight styles, you can wrap your hair using a wide tooth comb and then tie it up if that is what you prefer. Another topic of importance when it comes to the materials you use on your hair are the materials you use to style your hair. Some hair ties and headbands can be damaging to hair.

If you regularly wear cotton headbands, your hair can become damaged with regular use. If you can't live without a headband (some days I prefer to use one for an easy and cute style), make sure you use fabrics that won't damage the hair, such as satin or silk. If you absolutely must wear a headband made of cotton, make sure to generously moisturize the area where the headband will be, and don't make a habit of wearing cotton headbands regularly. If you regularly wear your hair in a ponytail, stay away from rubber bands; rubber bands cause split ends.

Once again, you should try to buy hair ties made of fabrics such as satin and silk, but if cotton is your only option (such as a cotton scrunchie) make sure that the hair tie doesn't fit too tight and make sure that your hair is moisturized a little more since it will be in contact with a fabric that will draw moisture away from your hair. If you regularly wear your hair down, the underside of your hair will need a little more moisture because it will be in contact with the back of your shirt for most of the day. Be mindful that the back of your shirt can cause damaging friction to your hair, so changing up your style can give your hair a break from the damage that it experiences every day.

Chapter 8: Chemically Altered Hair (Relaxed, Colored, Permed, or Texturized)

There are many women who choose not to keep their natural hair texture but still want to grow their hair long, thick, and healthy. Many believe that those who choose to straighten their hair are filled with self-hate, but this is not always the case. I believe that all women have a right to choose how they want their hair to look, and all women are beautiful: from relaxed to natural, it doesn't matter. There are many other reasons why a woman would choose to change the chemical composition of her hair, and they include ease of styling and fashion.

I will say this: natural hair is stronger than chemically altered hair; chemically altered hair is broken down in order to alter its texture or color. Make sure to follow the directions precisely on your chemical of choice, and never over-process your hair. When you reapply the chemical, make sure that you are only processing your new growth. I wouldn't recommend mixing chemicals (using a relaxer and color for example). The chances of your hair bouncing back from such harsh treatment are small.

Chemicals break down the proteins in the hair in order to alter its composition, so you need to replace these proteins. Like I discussed in the strengthening chapter, you can use gelatin to do this. I also strongly recommend using henna. Henna reinforces the proteins in the hair by clinging to them. People who chemically alter their hair will benefit even more from protein and henna treatments than people with natural hair. Your hair will need more strength. I recommend that those with chemically altered hair do a bi-weekly gelatin treatment and weekly henna treatment for the first month. Remember to follow your protein and henna treatments with a deep conditioning treatment every time. After a month, you should see an improvement in your hair. It should be stronger, more durable, and shed less. Then you can cut down to doing your gelatin and henna treatments to once a month.

More regular hair treatments is the price you pay for having chemically treated hair. Chemically treated hair needs extra care. Also consider that chemical treatments can make the hair more porous, so moisturizing the hair more regularly and using sealant oils will be a must. Henna can help lessen the porosity of the hair, so this is yet another benefit of doing more regular henna treatments.

You will also need to be gentler with the way you handle your hair. Be cognizant of this while combing and styling the hair. Many women who relax their hair tend to wash it less and use more heat on the hair than those with natural hair textures. The reason they do this is to preserve their style by any means necessary. If you must, keep your hair wrapped at night using a wide-toothed wooden comb in order to preserve your hairstyle for longer stretches of time.

I wouldn't recommend using heat on your hair more than twice a week in this situation, and you'll definitely need to get a good heat protector to minimize the damage to your already delicate hair. The more you use chemicals and heat on your hair, the more likely you are to create split ends. The ends of your hair will need special care if you choose to go this route. Keeping the ends of your hair thoroughly moisturized is a must. In order to see the maximum benefit of your hair growth efforts, you will need to minimize the damage, thus minimizing the need to cut your ends, which is the oldest part of your hair.

You do this by minimizing the heat and strain placed on the ends, handling them with care, replacing the protein that has been lost, and making sure your protective and moisturizing products are distributed thoroughly from the root to tip. If you follow the methods in this book plus the added tips provided in this chapter, there is no reason why you can't grow long, strong, healthy hair in spite of using chemicals on your hair.

Chapter 9: Caring For Your Hair Under Hair Extensions

I despise it when I hear people say that only women who hate themselves wear weaves. Even though I pride myself in having long healthy hair, I will personally wear a weave if I want to change my hair color or style temporarily. I look at weaves as I would an outfit, purse, or a pair of shoes. Wearing a weave can give you a needed break from styling your hair every day, and if it is taken care of properly, your hair can flourish. It is also another valid option if you plan to transition from relaxed to natural hair.

9-1: Choosing Your Hairstylist Wisely:

The first and most important step in keeping the hair healthy underneath a weave is to choose your stylist wisely. Once your hair is ruined, there is no turning back, so you must guard it as if you are guarding a valuable treasure. Be discerning about who you let style your hair. Ideally, it is best to choose someone who is knowledgeable about natural hair care as well as hair extensions.

The best way to identify a good hairdresser is through word of mouth and observation. I remember when I first visited Memphis and was in search of a local hairdresser. I found a promising hairdresser on Instagram and decided to give her a try. Upon meeting her, she was without her weave, and her real hair was damaged. I promptly made an excuse to cancel the appointment. Although she was talented in installing hair extensions, she apparently had no knowledge of caring for the hair underneath. It was not worth the risk to my natural hair.

If necessary, you may have to speak up to your hairdresser about the way that she/he handles your hair. You want your hairdresser to be gentle with your hair, combing it gently from the tips to the roots to remove tangles and being gentle while braiding your hair. I have seen many hairdressers, although good at styling weaves, that did not show proper care to the hair underneath and yanked away at it unnecessarily while prepping the style. You don't want a hairdresser who is okay with causing split ends with no regards to your real hair just to create a hairstyle. Yes, your extensions may be gorgeous, but your hair is suffering underneath. You may even need to bring your own comb to the salon because I still see many stylists using standard combs with seams.

9-2: Choosing Your Hairstyle Carefully:

If you choose to wear a weave and still plan to grow your real hair, you will need to be careful of the hairstyle that you choose. As a general rule, I stay away from any weave style that requires glue. My personal favorite is a sew-in with a lace closure. That way, my hair is braided underneath and I don't have to worry about applying constant heat to a leave out (hair that you leave out of the weave to cover and blend with the weave in order to make it look more natural). If you choose the correct hairdresser, a full closure sew-in with a lace part will look natural.

I have tried a net installation under my sew-ins in the past, and I found it too difficult to wash, dry, and moisturize my hair thoroughly underneath. I install three bundles of hair, and a net is not necessary for that amount. For that reason, I don't recommend them, as your hair and scalp's health should be of the upmost importance to you if you want to grow your hair long and healthy. A sew-in that is installed properly with good human hair can last up to three months. This can give your hair a much needed break from daily styling.

Another of my favorite protective styles is single box braids or Senegalese twists. These styles can last for up to three months on thick hair, depending on your new growth. Be careful if you have fine hair. If you have fine hair, I wouldn't leave these styles in for more than two months at the most. These styles can become too heavy and weigh fine hair down, and there's an added danger for fine hair with having twists because leaving them in too long can cause your hair to lock up (form dreadlocks). Whether you have fine hair or thick hair, you would need to get your edges re-braided or re-twisted once a month. This is because your new growth can cause the braids to weigh your hair down and pull your edges out.

9-3: How to Cleanse and Moisturize Your Hair Under Your Hair Extensions:

The good thing about hair extensions is that your hair will lie unbothered, having a break from daily abuse. This makes your job easier, as all you will have to do is make sure that your hair and scalp remain clean and moisturized and also that your scalp is fed the needed nutrients through your diet and topically. In the chapter about scalp health I go into detail on the needed nutrients for optimal hair growth. In the case of hair extensions, it can be bothersome to wash your hair twice a week, especially if your extensions are long.

For this reason, I would suggest washing your extensions once a week using shampoo and conditioner, making sure to rub the scalp and hair underneath while shampooing. Make sure to rinse the hair thoroughly, as shampoo and conditioner can seep into your braided hair underneath. This is the main reason why I don't like using the net; it is hard to wash your hair and scalp thoroughly. After washing, use a microfiber towel such as the Turbitwist to dry your hair as much as possible before sitting under a dryer.

I definitely recommend investing in a hair dryer that you can sit under at home. If you air dry your hair, you risk your braids underneath not drying properly, and it can cause your hair to smell spoiled. I've even heard extreme cases where the hair became mildewed underneath the weave because the person did not dry their hair properly and it remained moist. After the hair is completely dry, if you use a daily moisturizer, it is now the time to place the moisturizer on your scalp and on your braided hair underneath, making sure not to get it on your extensions, as most hair extensions will become weighed down with too much oil.

The following is another method that I use to cleanse my scalp and underlying hair without having to wash my extensions, as it can be a hassle to wash your extensions more than once a week; I use a spray bottle and place ten drops of lavender oil, ten drops of rosemary oil, and two drops of peppermint oil in water. I turn my hair upside down and spray between each track directly on the scalp, then I massage it into my braids. This moisture will invigorate and cleanse the hair and scalp between washes. You can also use an apple cider vinegar rinse in a spray bottle to cleanse the hair in this same manner with the added benefit of clarifying the hair and scalp.

Afterwards, you should sit under the dryer to make sure that your hair underneath dries completely, which won't take more than twenty minutes in most cases. Then you should proceed to moisturize the scalp and hair underneath, making sure not to get it on your extensions. You can use these same methods while wearing twists or braids by paying attention to your scalp and new growth during the duration of your hairstyle. After you remove the style, give your hair a break for at least a week before getting a new one. Do your protein, henna, and moisturizing treatments at least a couple of days before you get a new weave style put in. If you follow these tips, there is no reason why your hair won't grow and be healthy while using these protective styles.

Chapter 10: Closing

I hope everyone enjoyed reading this information as much as I enjoyed sharing it with you. All of the information involves minor changes that can be easily implemented yet yield huge results. It's really as simple as changing a few things in your hair care regimen to get the hair of your dreams. Most importantly, it's not as expensive as you would think to have your dream hair. Instead of feeling that you are doomed to the land of unhealthy or short hair, you now have the knowledge that you need to successfully get over your hair hump.

Diagram 2.1: The Hair Bulb, The Hair Follicle, and the Oil Gland

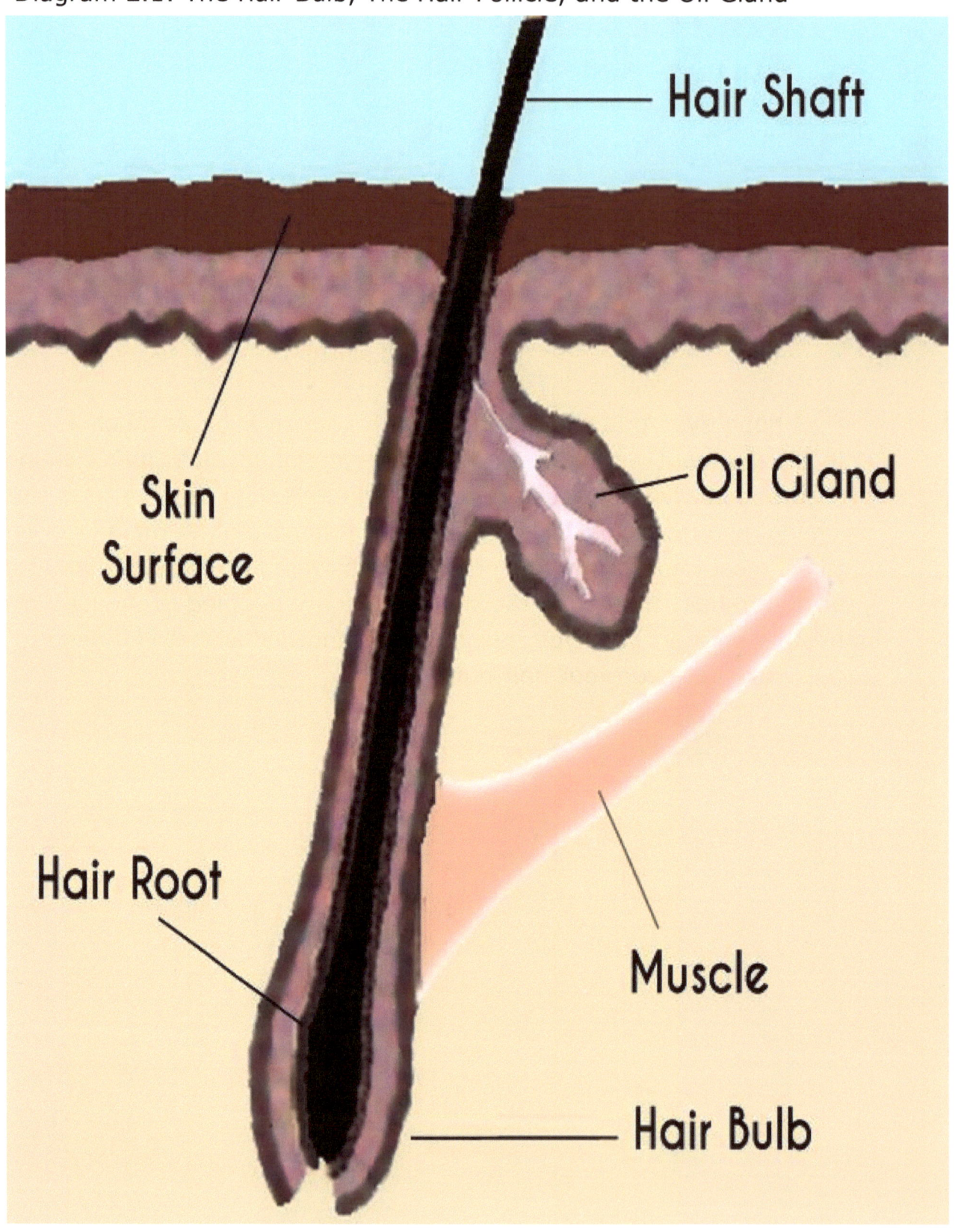

Diagram 2.2: The Three Layers of the Hair Shaft

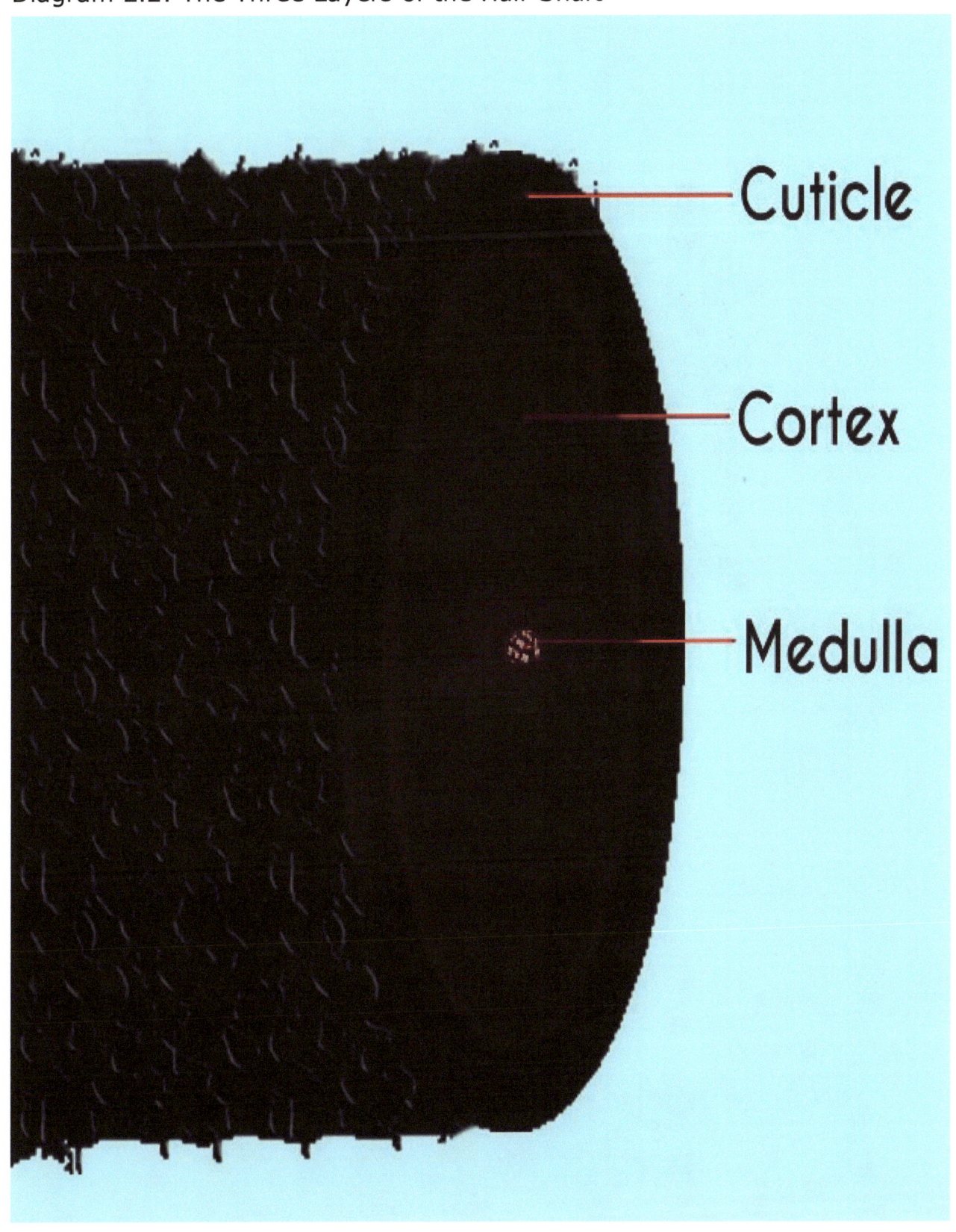

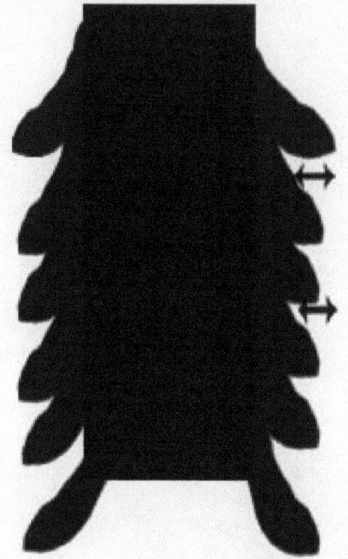

CLOSED CUTICLE

OPEN CUTICLE

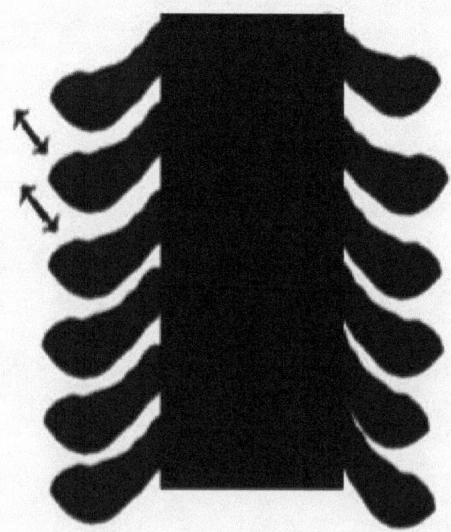

Diagram 5.1: Water Hardness in the U.S.

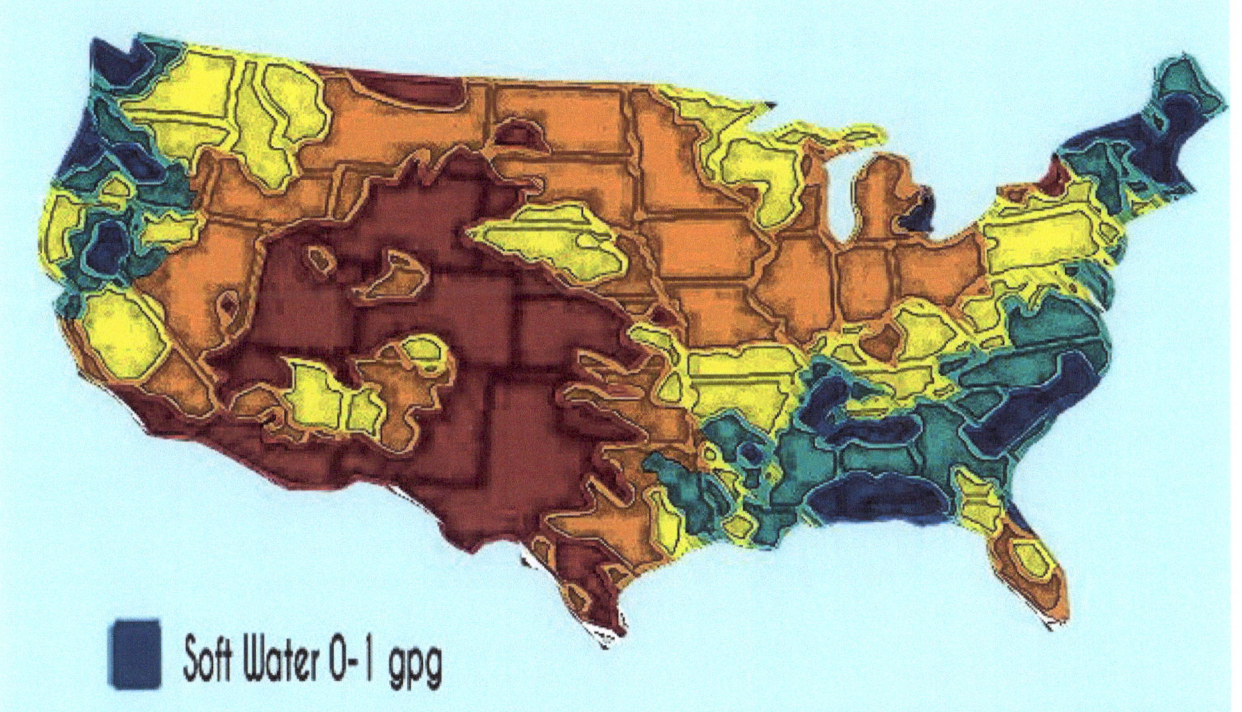

Soft Water 0-1 gpg

Slightly Hard Water: 1-3.5 gpg

Moderately Hard Water: 3.5-7 gpg

Hard Water: 7-10.5 gpg

Very Hard Water: Over 10.5 gpg

CONCENTRATION OF WATER HARDNESS IN GRAINS PER GALLON

Diagram 7.2: Comb Seam

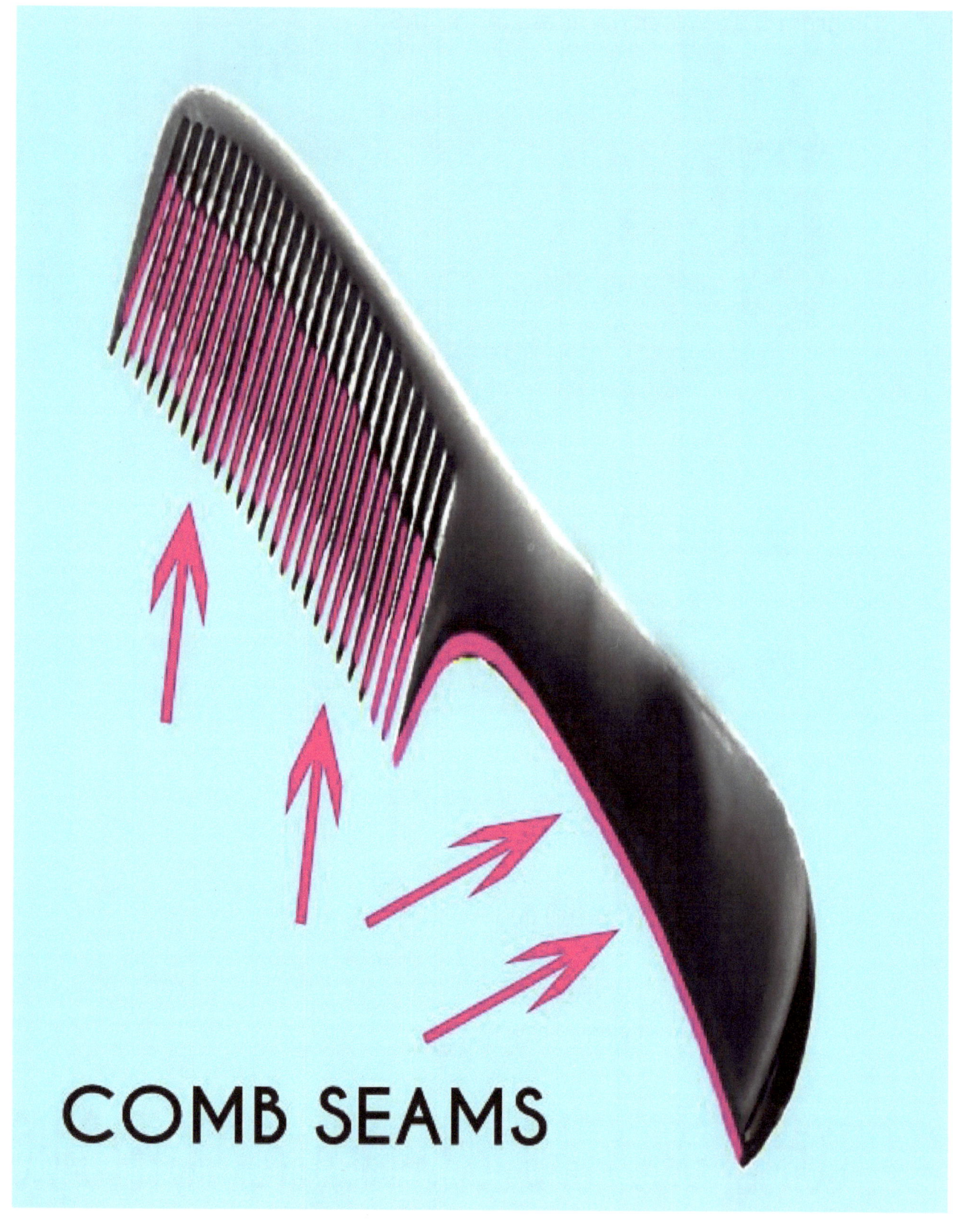

COMB SEAMS

Diagram 7.4: Healthy End Compared to a Split End

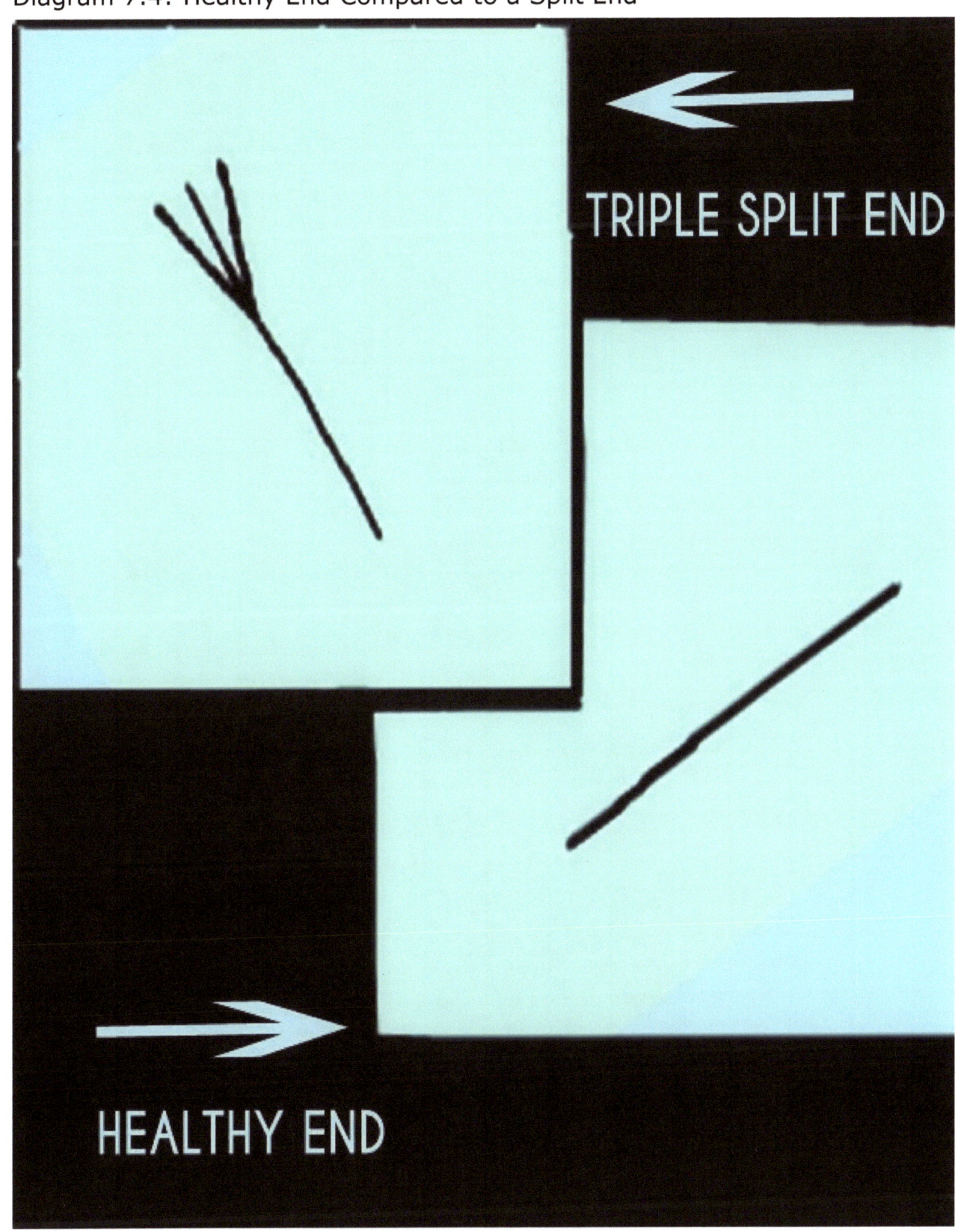

www.ingramcontent.com/pod-product-compliance
Lightning Source LLC
Chambersburg PA
CBHW041509280526
45792CB00004B/1185